THE GLOBAL IMPACT OF HEPATITIS E VIRUS

Steve k. Bryant

Copyright

Copyright © 2024 by **Steve k. Bryant**

Contents

Introduction

Hepatitis E Virus Overview (HEV)

One of the main causes of acute viral hepatitis worldwide is the RNA virus known as the hepatitis E virus (HEV), which is a member of the Hepeviridae family. The fecal-oral pathway is the main means of virus transmission, which frequently involves consuming tainted food or water. Even while HEV isn't as well-known as other hepatitis viruses like hepatitis B or C, it poses a serious threat to public health, especially in developing nations with poor water and sanitation infrastructure.

There are multiple genotypes of HEV, with genotypes 1 and 2 being the most common in humans and found in Asia, Africa, and Latin America. Large waterborne outbreaks are caused by these genotypes. Conversely, genotypes 3 and 4 are zoonotic, meaning they harm both people and animals; they are typically seen in industrialized nations. Consumption of raw or undercooked meat from infected animals, including pig, deer, and shellfish, is frequently associated with these genotypes.

HEV infection can cause severe hepatitis, which can be fatal, especially in pregnant women and those with underlying liver diseases. Alternatively, the infection might show clinically as silent. Particularly in the third trimester of pregnancy, when the death rate might exceed 25%, the virus can cause fulminant hepatic failure. Extrahepatic symptoms of HEV, such as neurological problems, renal dysfunction, and hematological abnormalities, have been increasingly documented in recent years.

Studying HEV in Connection with the Swine Industry and Reproductive Health Is Important

Sexual and Reproductive Health

Because of the serious effects that HEV can have on expectant mothers, research on the relationship between the virus and reproductive health is essential. Due to immune system changes brought on by pregnancy, women are more vulnerable to serious consequences from a variety of illnesses, including HEV. The virus can cause serious fetal outcomes such miscarriage, stillbirth, and preterm delivery in addition to significant maternal morbidity and mortality. It is essential to comprehend the pathways through which HEV impacts pregnancy in order to create focused interventions that will safeguard this susceptible group.

Furthermore, recent studies have started to shed light on the possible effects of HEV on the health of male reproduction. According to studies, HEV can exist in semen and may have an impact on the motility and quality of sperm, which could result in infertility. Given the significance of reproductive health to both individual and society well-being, this presents serious public health implications. Further research into these impacts may shed light on male infertility and lead to novel approaches to diagnosis and therapy.

Pork Sector

The effect of HEVs on the swine sector is an additional crucial factor that needs careful examination. Pigs are thought to be a major source of HEV, especially the human-infecting genotypes 3 and 4. The methods used by the swine business, particularly the extensive use of artificial insemination, can make it easier for HEV to spread through contaminated semen. Because of the virus's potential for zoonotic transmission, this puts human health at risk in addition to animal health.

There are substantial economic ramifications for the pork sector. Even while HEV rarely results in overt clinical disease in pigs, subclinical infections can nonetheless have an impact on reproductive health and output. Effective screening and management techniques are required to address the worry that HEV may have an adverse influence on the general health of herds and the effectiveness of pig breeding operations.

In addition, the fact that pigs can transmit HEV to humans—especially when contaminated meat is consumed—underlines the necessity of thorough food safety protocols. In order to ensure the health of both animals and the general people, it can be helpful to identify crucial control points for the HEV virus by researching it in relation to the swine business.

The book's objectives and scope

With an emphasis on the effects of HEV on swine production and reproductive health, this book attempts to offer a thorough analysis of the disease. The following are the book's goals:

To Offer a Comprehensive Understanding of HEV

Describe in detail the clinical signs, epidemiology, and virology of HEV.

Examine the various HEV genotypes, their geographic distribution, and their modes of transmission.

To Investigate HEV's Effect on Reproductive Health

Examine the impact of HEV on expectant mothers, as well as the pathways that result in unfavorable results.

Examine the new data that connects HEV to male infertility and consider the possible mechanisms at play.

Talk about the wider effects of HEV on reproductive health and possible remedies.

To Investigate the Connection Between the Swine Industry and HEV

Examine the frequency of HEV in pig populations and the effects it has on the well-being and output of swine.

Analyze the possibility that artificial insemination and other breeding techniques could spread the HEV virus.

Analyze HEV's zoonotic potential and its effects on public health and food safety.

To Determine Prevention and Control Strategies for HEVs

Examine the most recent approaches to preventing and managing HEV in animal and human populations.

Make recommendations based on data to enhance HEV control in the swine sector.

Emphasize the necessity of using interdisciplinary methods to solve the problems that HEV presents.

To Promote HEV Knowledge and Research

Educate the public, lawmakers, veterinary professionals, and healthcare providers about HEV.

Promote more HEV research, especially in the fields of swine agriculture and reproductive health.

lays the groundwork for next research and the creation of policy intended to lessen the effects of HEVs.

Organization of the Book

The book is structured into four primary sections, each of which focuses on a distinct HEV topic

Section I: Comprehending the Hepatitis E Virus

This section covers the virology, epidemiology, and transmission mechanisms of HEV to give readers a basic grasp of the virus. It establishes the context for the talks that follow about how the virus affects pig health and reproduction.

section II: HEV and Reproductive Health

The precise consequences of HEV on reproductive health are covered in detail in this section. It looks at the serious consequences of HEV infection in expectant mothers and the growing body of research that connects HEV to infertility in males. The aim is to present a thorough overview of the possible processes and ways that HEV may impact reproductive health.

Section III: The Swine Industry's Use of HEVs

The effect of HEVs on the swine sector is the main topic of this section. It evaluates the dangers of artificial insemination, the prevalence of HEV in pigs, and the larger effects on animal productivity and health. There is also discussion of HEV's zoonotic potential and how it may affect food safety.

Section IV: Wider Consequences of HEV

The topic of HEV's wider effects outside the swine industry and reproductive health is covered in this concluding part. It discusses the present state of public health and policy responses to extrahepatic symptoms of HEV, including neurological and pancreatic problems. A review of prospective approaches for HEV control and prevention as well as future research directions round out this part.

In summary

The hepatitis E virus is a serious yet frequently disregarded infection that has a wide range of effects on animal and human health. Its effect on reproductive health, especially in expectant mothers and maybe in men, emphasizes the need for a more thorough comprehension of the virus's methods of action. Further highlighting the connection between animal and human health and the significance of a One Health approach to disease control is the function of HEV in the swine industry.

The goal of this book is to close the information gap by offering a thorough analysis of HEV, covering everything from its fundamental biology to its intricate relationships with both human and animal hosts. Through an examination of the complex effects of HEV, the book aims to educate readers and motivate action to lessen the virus's impact and eventually enhance animal and human health.

SECTION I

Comprehending the Hepatitis E Virus

Chapter 1

Definition of the Hepatitis E Virus.

The Origins and History of HEV

After several hepatitis epidemics in Asia, the hepatitis E virus (HEV) was discovered for the first time in the early 1980s. Many cases of what is now known as hepatitis E were previously categorized as non-A, non-B hepatitis before its identification. These cases were classified as a unique, if poorly understood, form of hepatitis as they did not match the characteristics of either hepatitis A or hepatitis B, the only two known hepatitis viruses at the time.

Russian virologist Dr. Mikhail Balayan is credited with discovering HEV in 1981 while looking into a hepatitis outbreak in the former Soviet Union. Balayan discovered the virus was the cause of the outbreak. In order to better understand the infection process, Balayan and his colleagues took samples from afflicted people and, in a controversial move, swallowed a fecal suspension made from these samples. By utilizing electron microscopy to successfully identify the virus particles in their own stool samples, this self-experimentation resulted in the first image of the HEV virion.

Subsequent studies conducted in the 1980s and 1990s confirmed HEV's status as a unique virus after this original discovery. The sequencing of the viral genome was made possible by developments in molecular biology techniques, which improved our knowledge of the structure and classification of the virus. HEV was acknowledged as a serious public health risk by the early 1990s, especially in areas with inadequate sanitation and hygiene standards.

The composition and categorization of HEVs

With a single-stranded positive-sense RNA genome that is roughly 7.2 kilobases long, HEV is a tiny, non-enveloped virus. Three open reading frames (ORFs) make up the genome: ORF1, ORF2, and ORF3. These ORFs encode proteins necessary for the infection and replication processes of the virus.

Non-structural proteins involved in viral replication, such as helicase, protease, methyltransferase, and RNA-dependent RNA polymerase (RdRp), are encoded by ORF1.

The capsid protein, which makes up the outer shell of the virus and is essential for both immune response elicitation and infectivity, is encoded by ORF2.

A tiny, multifunctional protein that is encoded by ORF3 is involved in both viral egress and host cell signaling pathway regulation.

The Hepeviridae family, which is further subdivided into the genera Orthohepevirus and Piscihepevirus, is where HEV is categorized. There are four species in the Orthohepevirus genus, which includes Orthohepevirus A, B, C, and D, and is mostly relevant to infections in humans and mammals.

The HEV genotypes 1 through 4—which are the most pertinent to human health—are included in orthohepevirus A.

Genotype 1 is limited to human hosts and is primarily prevalent in Asia and Africa.

Although it is less prevalent, genotype 2 has been linked to epidemics in Africa and Mexico.

With a wide geographic range that includes Europe, North America, and Asia, genotype 3 can infect both people and animals, most commonly pigs.

Mainly found in Asia, genotype 4 has the ability to spread zoonotically, meaning it can infect both people and animals.

In birds, orthohepevirus B is present.

Rodents and ferrets are infected with orthohepevirus C.

Bats are infected with orthohepevirus D.

The categorization of HEV genotypes is essential in comprehending the dynamics of virus transmission, epidemiology, and possible zoonotic reservoirs.

Epidemiology and Worldwide Dispersion

With 20 million infections and 70,000 fatalities from HEV each year, it is one of the leading causes of acute viral hepatitis globally. Because of variables including food habits, water quality, and sanitation, its epidemiology differs greatly between areas.

Distribution and Transmission of the HEV Genotype

Genotypes 1 and 2: Contaminated water sources are frequently the means by which these genotypes are mainly spread through feces. They are widespread in areas of Asia, Africa, and Central America with inadequate sanitary facilities. Big outbreaks are frequently linked to occurrences that affect the quality of the water, such as monsoon rains. Humans are the usual hosts of infection, and there are no notable animal repositories for these genotypes.

Genotypes 3 and 4: Because they are zoonotic, these genotypes have a more complicated epidemiology. Both human and animal populations contain them; the main reservoirs are domestic pigs and wild boars. Eating raw or undercooked meat from infected animals, especially pork products, can expose humans to illnesses. While genotype 4 is primarily found in Asia, genotype 3 is more common in developed regions like North America, Europe, and some parts of Asia. Occupational exposure is another factor that increases the incidence of these genotypes, as seen in farmers and veterinarians.

Localized Epidemiology

Asia: Especially with regard to Genotypes 1 and 4, Asia has the highest incidence of HEV infections. Large epidemics are regularly reported from nations including Bangladesh, Pakistan, China, India, and others. High rates of pregnancy-related death are seen during these epidemics, which are frequently connected to contaminated water supplies. Undercooked pork and wild animal consumption are also frequently linked to Genotype 4 infections in China and Japan.

Africa: The most common genotype of HEV is Genotype 1, and the disease poses a serious threat to public health there. In areas like Sudan, Uganda, and Chad that have inadequate sanitation, outbreaks happen often. Humanitarian situations that put a burden on the water and sanitation systems currently in place, like refugee movements and hostilities, frequently make these outbreaks worse.

Europe and North America: These two regions are more likely to experience isolated instances of HEV than significant epidemics. The most prevalent genotype is genotype 3, and illnesses are frequently associated with eating undercooked pork products or coming into close contact with pigs. Despite being less common than in Asia and Africa, HEV is becoming more widespread here, which emphasizes the significance of keeping an eye on zoonotic transmission.

Central and South America: Mexico has reported significant outbreaks of HEV Genotypes 1 and 2, which are found in Central America. HEV is not as well understood in South America, yet isolated reports of Genotype 3 cases suggest zoonotic transmission exists there.

Risk Elements and At-Risk Groups

Some demographics are more vulnerable to HEV infection and serious illness consequences:

Pregnant Women: The danger of severe HEV infection is much higher in pregnant women, especially in the third trimester, when fatality rates can exceed 25%. Although the exact causes of this increased vulnerability are unknown, it is thought that pregnancy-related changes in hormone and immune systems impact the body's ability to fight off the virus.

People with Pre-existing Liver Disease: Individuals who have cirrhosis or co-infections of hepatitis B and C are more vulnerable to serious consequences from HEV infection. In some people, the extra liver damage brought on by HEV may result in abrupt liver failure.

Elderly and Immunocompromised Individuals: Individuals in their latter years and those with weaker immune systems, such as organ transplant recipients and chemotherapy patients, are more vulnerable to long-term HEV infection, especially when it comes to Genotype 3.

In these groups, chronic infection can result in cirrhosis and progressive liver disease.

Control and Preventive Actions

HEV prevention and control that is effective must take a multimodal approach that addresses reservoirs in both humans and animals. Important tactics consist of:

Enhancing Sanitation and Water Quality: It's critical to provide access to clean water and sanitation facilities in areas where HEV is spread through contaminated water. Additionally effective in lowering transmission are public health efforts that encourage proper cleanliness.

Food Safety Practices: It's critical to inform the public about the dangers of eating raw or undercooked meat, especially pork. Making sure animal products are cooked properly can stop HEV Genotypes 3 and 4 from spreading zoonotically.

Immunization: Although a vaccine (HEV 239) has been created and granted a license in China, it is not yet generally accessible around the world. The HEV vaccination might be made more widely available, particularly in high-risk locations, to drastically lower the disease burden.

Screening and Surveillance: Putting in place screening initiatives for high-risk groups including organ transplant patients and pregnant women can aid in the early detection and treatment of HEV infections. Additionally, improved surveillance systems are better able to track and contain outbreaks.

Veterinary Interventions: Biosecurity measures and maybe HEV vaccinations for pigs could lower the danger of zoonotic transmission in the swine sector. Controlling the spread both within and between farms can also be aided by routinely testing pig herds for HEV.

A thorough examination of the Hepatitis E Virus's (HEV) structure, history, epidemiology, and categorization is necessary to comprehend the virus. Considerable progress has been made in our understanding of the virus and its effects on world health since its discovery in the early 1980s. The extensive geographic distribution and variety of HEV's transmission channels underscore how difficult it is to contain this infection. The necessity for specialized public health initiatives to lessen the burden of HEV is highlighted by the disparities in epidemiological patterns seen between genotypes and geographical areas. The precise effects of HEV on swine production and reproductive health will be covered in more detail in the upcoming chapters, which will offer a comprehensive overview of this important public health issue.

Chapter 2

Mechanisms of Transmission and Infection

Transmission Modes

There are several ways that the hepatitis E virus (HEV) can spread, which adds to its broad prevalence and varied epidemiological patterns. For the purpose of creating efficient preventative and control measures, it is essential to comprehend these transmission channels. Fecal-oral, zoonotic, and possibly sexual transmission are the main means of transmission.

Fecal-Oral Transmission

The most well-established method of HEV transmission, especially for genotypes 1 and 2, is the fecal-oral pathway. This method usually entails consuming food or water tainted with the virus-containing feces.

Waterborne epidemics: When HEV contaminates water supplies in unsanitary locations, it can result in significant epidemics. Events such as intense downpours, floods, or malfunctions in water treatment facilities can set off these outbreaks. Some notable instances are the extensive HEV outbreaks in Africa and India, when the main infection vectors were found to be tainted drinking water supplies.

Foodborne Transmission: HEV transmission can also occur through contaminated food. This is particularly relevant in areas where food preparation hygiene standards are inadequate. Even while outbreaks caused by water are increasingly frequent, foodborne transmission is still a major risk factor.

Person-to-Person Transmission: Direct transmission between individuals through the fecal-oral pathway is uncommon but nevertheless feasible, particularly in unsanitary environments. This mode is more prevalent in homes or among a close friend or relative of an afflicted person.

Transmission of Zoonotic Organisms

Zoonotic transmission, which is the process by which the virus spreads from animals to people, is mostly linked to genotypes 3 and 4. There are animal reservoirs for these genotypes, with domestic pigs and wild boars being the main donors.

Animal Reservoirs: Pigs are the main animal reservoir for HEV genotypes 3 and 4. Worldwide, pig populations are endemic to the virus, which is very prevalent in both farmed and wild pig populations. There is a chance that the virus could infect people in other animals like deer and rabbits.

Eating Contaminated Meat: Eating raw or undercooked meat from sick animals is the most frequent way that zoonotic diseases are spread. Pork products are specifically mentioned, with foods like liver sausages and uncooked or barely cooked pork offering serious health concerns. Instances and outbreaks connected to food practices have been documented in the US, France, Japan, and other nations.

Occupational Exposure: Those with intimate contact with animals, such as farmers, veterinarians, and abattoir workers, are more likely to contract HEV infection from the animals themselves or from animal products.

Seroconversion and symptomatic or asymptomatic infections are possible outcomes of these occupational exposures.

Possibility of Sexual Transmission

Although zoonotic and fecal-oral transmissions are well known, new research indicates that HEV may also be sexually transferred, especially through semen. The ramifications of this form of transmission for disease prevention and reproductive health make it extremely interesting, even though it has not been fully established.

Semen: Research has shown that HEV RNA can be found in the semen of infected people, suggesting that the virus can be excreted in seminal fluid. Although the effectiveness and frequency of this route of transmission are yet unclear, this finding suggests the possibility of sexual transmission.

Implications for Reproductive Health: The management of reproductive health as well as the spread of HEV in populations may be significantly impacted if sexual transmission is proven. It may be crucial to concentrate on detecting HEV in semen donors and comprehending how HEV affects fertility.

HEV Lifecycle in Animals and Humans

HEVs go through multiple stages in their life cycle, including entrance into the host, replication, and shedding. It is essential to comprehend this lifecycle in order to pinpoint possible intervention sites that could stop the spread of the illness and lower its impact.

Access and Primary Infection

Human Hosts: Human Ebola virus (HEV) enters the human body by contaminated food or water consumption, or maybe through sex-related contact with semen. The virus enters the circulation after passing from the stomach and into the small intestine, where it penetrates the intestinal epithelium.

Contaminated feed or water is usually how the virus enters animals, especially pigs. Like in humans, the virus enters the body through the intestinal barrier and spreads throughout the bloodstream.

Duplication

Liver Infection: The liver is the main location where HEV replication occurs. Hepatocytes are the cells of the liver where the virus replicates. Non-structural proteins (encoded by ORF1) required for viral replication are produced by translation of the viral RNA genome. A complementary negative-sense RNA strand is created during the replication process, and this strand is subsequently used as a template to create new positive-sense RNA genomes.

Assembly and Release: Recently manufactured viral genomes are enclosed in capsids, which are made of entire virions and are encoded by ORF2. Following their release from hepatocytes into the bile, these virions are eventually expelled in the stools. This excrement leakage promotes the fecal-oral transmission pathway. Furthermore, some virions are discharged into the bloodstream, which heightens the risk of viremia and its dissemination to other organs.

Transmission and Shedding

Human Hosts: One of the most important stages of HEV transmission in people is the shedding of HEV in feces. Acute infection is characterized by a peak viral load, which can be excreted by infected persons for several weeks. New illnesses can then arise from contaminated food or drink.

Animal Hosts: HEV is excreted in pig feces in a manner similar to humans, contaminating the environment and possibly spreading to humans or other pigs. The virus may also be found in the meat of animals that have been affected, putting human health at risk.

Infections That Are Symptomatic vs. Asymptomatic

HEV infections can exhibit a broad range of clinical symptoms, from individuals with no symptoms to those with severe symptoms. The complicated interplay of host immunological status, virus genotype, and underlying medical problems determines the severity of HEV infection.

infections without symptoms

Prevalence: Infections with no symptoms are frequent, especially in areas where they are endemic. Research has demonstrated that a sizable percentage of HEV infections, particularly those brought on by genotypes 3 and 4, do not generate any discernible symptoms. Studies that identify antibodies against HEV in populations, known as seroprevalence studies, frequently show a high incidence of prior infection in the absence of symptoms.

immunological Reaction: Most asymptomatic infections trigger an immunological reaction strong enough to eradicate the virus without seriously harming the liver. Antibodies are a sign of prior exposure and immunity, albeit the strength and longevity of this immunity can differ.

Implications for Public Health: The virus can still spread throughout a community even among carriers who show no symptoms. The silent transmission of diseases can make it more difficult to contain epidemics since people may unintentionally contaminate the environment and spread the disease

Manifest Infections

Acute Hepatitis: The severity of acute hepatitis caused by symptomatic HEV infections can vary. Jaundice, exhaustion, nausea, vomiting, abdominal discomfort, and fever are typical symptoms. Acute HEV usually has a self-limiting clinical course that ends in a few of weeks to months.

Severe Outcomes: Severe sickness is more likely to strike certain populations. Fulminant hepatitis, which is characterized by rapid liver failure and a high death rate, can strike pregnant women, especially in the third trimester of pregnancy. Severe consequences and liver decompensation are also more likely in people with pre-existing liver diseases, such as chronic hepatitis B or C.

Chronic Infections: Although acute infections are more common, immunocompromised people—such as organ transplant recipients, cancer patients, and HIV/AIDS patients—can develop chronic HEV infections. If left untreated, chronic HEV can cause cirrhosis and liver failure due to its persistent viremia and liver inflammation. The most frequent association with genotype 3 is persistent infections.

Factors Affecting the Results of Infectio

A number of variables affect the occurrence and intensity of symptoms in the event that a HEV infection manifests as symptoms, including:

Viral Genotype: The degree of virulence varies throughout HEV genotypes. Large outbreaks and symptomatic sickness are more likely to be caused by genotypes 1 and 2, especially in areas with inadequate sanitation. Zoonotic genotypes 3 and 4 are frequently linked to lesser forms of the disease, but in susceptible groups, they can have serious consequences.

Host Immune Status: The host's immune state is a major factor in deciding how a HEV infection turns out. People with strong immune systems have a higher chance of overcoming the virus and experiencing a minimal or painless illness. Conversely, those with impaired immune systems are more vulnerable to severe illness and persistent infections.

Pregnancy: Women who are expecting, especially in the third trimester, are at a heightened risk of developing a severe HEV infection, which frequently results in fulminant hepatitis and high fatality rates. Although the precise mechanisms causing this elevated risk are not fully known, changes in hormones and the immune system during pregnancy may be involved.

Age and Comorbidities: Severe HEV infection is more common in older adults, those with pre-existing liver disease, and those with other comorbid diseases. The virus may have a more severe effect as a result of comorbidities and age-related decreases in immune function.

Hepatitis E virus (HEV) infection and transmission methods are intricate and multidimensional, encompassing fecal-oral, zoonotic, and even sexual pathways. The HEV lifecycle illustrates the several phases at which interventions can be put in place to stop the virus's spread, from entry and replication to shedding and transmission. The variety of clinical presentations, ranging from infections with no symptoms to those with severe symptoms, emphasizes the necessity for a comprehensive knowledge of the variables affecting infection outcomes. We can create focused initiatives to lessen the impact of HEV and safeguard vulnerable groups by clarifying these mechanisms. These next few chapters will go into further detail.

SECTION II

HEV and Reproductive Health in

Chapter 3

Pregnancy and HEV

HEV's Effect on Expectant Mothers

For expectant mothers, the hepatitis E virus (HEV) poses a serious health danger, particularly in areas where the virus is endemic. HEV infection can have serious consequences for pregnant women, with the third trimester carrying the greatest risk. HEV can have a significant negative effect on pregnancy, increasing the risk of morbidity and death for both the mother and the fetus.

Increased Susceptibility: Pregnant women are more vulnerable to infections, including HEV, due to a number of physiological changes brought on by pregnancy that may impact the immune system. Pregnancy-related hormonal changes may affect immunological responses and reduce the body's capacity to develop a strong defense against viral infections. Pregnant women's greater susceptibility to HEV infections is believed to be influenced by this weakened immune system.

Severe Liver Disease: Fulminant hepatitis, a rapid and severe form of liver failure, is a much higher risk for pregnant women infected with HEV. The hallmark of fulminant hepatitis is abrupt liver cell death, which results in the loss of liver function. Jaundice, coagulopathy (disorders of bleeding), encephalopathy (dysfunction of the brain), and multi-organ failure are among the symptoms. When fulminant hepatitis E is present in pregnancy, the death rate can be as high as 25%, particularly in the third trimester.

Obstetric issues: Preterm labor, intrauterine fetal mortality, and stillbirth are just a few of the obstetric issues that can result from HEV infection during pregnancy. Severe hepatitis's stress and inflammation might induce early labor, endangering the newborn's health. Furthermore, the virus has the ability to pass across the placenta, infecting the fetus and causing negative consequences like fetal discomfort and death.

Vertical Transmission: Although the precise processes underlying the vertical transmission of HEV from mother to fetus are still unclear, it has been established. It appears that HEV can get across the placental barrier because the virus is present in the placenta, amniotic fluid, and fetal tissues. Babies born to moms infected with HEV may have potentially fatal acute hepatitis or other delivery problems.

Risk Factors for Pregnancy Deaths Associated with HEV

In areas where HEV is endemic, the effects on pregnancy are very severe. Pregnant women in these places have high death rates due to a number of factors:

Healthcare Infrastructure: In many impoverished nations, there is insufficient infrastructure for treating severe HEV infection patients. Pregnant women with fulminant hepatitis E who have limited access to advanced medical care, such as intensive care units (ICUs) and liver transplantation facilities, are at increased risk of fatality.

Malnutrition and Coinfections: In addition to experiencing infectious disorders and malnutrition, pregnant women living in endemic areas may also have additional illnesses that compromise their immune systems. In certain regions, illnesses including malaria, HIV/AIDS, and other parasite diseases are prevalent and can exacerbate HEV infection.

Delayed Diagnosis and Treatment: In environments with low resources, diagnostic facilities and awareness are often lacking, leading to delays in diagnosis and treatment. It's possible that pregnant women who exhibit jaundice and liver dysfunction don't receive a timely diagnosis of HEV, which could cause delays in supportive treatment and appropriate management.

High Viral Load: Research indicates that HEV-positive pregnant women frequently have greater viral loads than non-pregnant people. Higher viral loads are linked to worsening symptoms and less favorable results. Although the exact causes of this enhanced viral replication in pregnant women are unknown, the changed immunological milieu that results from pregnancy may be one of them.

Case Studies and Data from Epidemiology

The serious effects of HEV on expectant mothers are demonstrated by a plethora of case studies and epidemiological data. These examples offer insightful information about the clinical presentation, results, and difficulties in managing HEV during pregnancy.

Case Study No. 1: India

One of the nations most impacted by HEV is India, where tainted water supplies are frequently the cause of outbreaks. Pregnant women have been affected by a number of HEV outbreaks, with concerning fatality rates, according to a New Delhi study.

Outbreak Description: The following describes an outbreak that occurred in 2008, Pregnant women had a disproportionately high rate of HEV infection as compared to the general population, according to a public health investigation. A major metropolitan community's use of tainted water was identified as the source of the outbreak.

Clinical Results: Jaundice, coagulopathy, and encephalopathy were among the severe symptoms that pregnant women infected with HEV showed. Pregnant women had a mortality rate of over 20%, with the third trimester accounting for the majority of deaths. Preterm labor and multiple occurrences of intrauterine fetal mortality were also documented.

Management Challenges: Managing instances of fulminant hepatitis was made extremely difficult by the dearth of liver transplantation facilities and intensive care units. Although many women received supportive care, the results were not as good because of the scarce resources and the delayed diagnosis.

Case Study No. 2 in Bangladesh

Pregnant women in Bangladesh, another nation with a high prevalence of HEV, have had multiple cases of problems connected to HEV documented. A retrospective study carried out in a Dhaka tertiary care hospital shed light on the clinical traits and results of pregnant women with HEV infection.

Study Population: Over the course of five years, 50 pregnant women with HEV diagnoses were included in the study. When these ladies were diagnosed, most of them were in the third trimester.

Clinical Presentation: Frequent signs and symptoms included vomiting, fever, jaundice, and stomach pain. Severe liver dysfunction was indicated by laboratory results showing high liver enzymes, elevated bilirubin levels, and prolonged clotting times.

Maternal and Fetal Outcomes: Fulminant hepatitis was the primary cause of death, with a reported 16% maternal mortality rate. Among the unfavorable fetal outcomes were stillbirth, low birth weight, and premature delivery. Acute hepatitis was the presenting symptom in afflicted newborns, and the estimated vertical transmission rate was 10%.

Implications for Public Health: The study emphasized the need for better treatment and diagnostic approaches to address HEV during pregnancy. The importance of public health programs aimed at enhancing sanitation and water quality as preventative measures against future epidemics was also emphasized.

Case Study No. 3 in Sudan

HEV is endemic in Sudan and presents a serious risk to expectant mothers. Important information on the epidemiology and effects of HEV on maternal health was obtained from an outbreak investigation carried out in a remote area of Sudan.

Investigation of the Outbreak: In 2014, a HEV outbreak happened in a remote area with little access to medical treatment and clean water. More than a thousand people were impacted by the outbreak, and a sizable fraction of those afflicted were pregnant women.

Clinical findings: Severe jaundice, coagulopathy, and encephalopathy were observed in pregnant women infected with HEV. An estimate of 30% was given for the rate of maternal mortality, with the third trimester accounting for the majority of deaths. Numerous occurrences of neonatal hepatitis and intrauterine fetal mortality were also reported by the inquiry.

Obstacles and Suggestions: In order to stop future HEV epidemics, better water and sanitation infrastructure is needed, as the pandemic made clear. The report suggested that focused public health initiatives be put into place, such as immunization drives for expectant mothers and the creation of referral facilities with the capacity to handle severe HEV cases.

Data from Epidemiology

Additional evidence of the serious effects of HEV on pregnant women is provided by epidemiological data from different locations. These data are crucial for determining the extent of the issue and directing public health initiatives.

Global Burden: According to estimates from the World Health Organization (WHO), HEV accounts for about 20 million infections and 70,000 fatalities globally each year. An important share of these deaths are pregnant women, especially in underdeveloped nations. The high rates of pregnancy-related mortality highlight the critical need for focused treatments.

Regional Differences: There are significant regional differences in the burden of HEV. HEV is a significant public health concern in Asia and Africa, where genotypes 1 and 2 are more common. Outbreaks in these areas frequently correlate with monsoon seasons or other circumstances that affect the quality of the water. On the other hand, HEV mostly generates sporadic instances associated with zoonotic transmission in developed regions like Europe and North America, where genotypes 3 and 4 are more prevalent.

Vaccination and Prevention: A useful tool for preventing HEV infection has been made possible by the development of the HEV vaccine (HEV 239) in China. The safety and effectiveness of the vaccine in preventing HEV infection, particularly in high-risk populations like pregnant women, have been proven by clinical trials. But the vaccination isn't yet generally accessible everywhere in the world. Increased availability of the HEV vaccination, especially in areas where it is endemic, may considerably lower the incidence of HEV during pregnancy.

Pregnant women are at serious risk from the Hepatitis E Virus (HEV), which can cause potentially fatal pregnancy problems. Pregnant women are especially vulnerable to severe HEV infection because of their weakened immune systems, changed physiology, and elevated virus loads. The substantial effects of HEV on maternal and fetal health are demonstrated by case studies from Sudan, Bangladesh, and India, underscoring the necessity of better preventive, therapeutic, and diagnostic approaches. The global burden of HEV in pregnancy is further highlighted by epidemiological statistics, which emphasizes the need for focused public health initiatives including immunization, greater sanitation, and upgraded healthcare facilities. In order to provide readers a thorough grasp of this important public health issue, the upcoming chapters will examine the wider effects of HEV on swine production and reproductive health.

Chapter 4

HEV and Male Infertility

Relationship between Male Infertility and HEV

Although acute liver disease has long been linked to the hepatitis E virus (HEV), new research indicates that the virus may also have an effect on male reproductive health. Male infertility affects millions of couples globally and is a serious public health concern. HEV and male infertility may be related, which is a new and significant field of study with consequences for public health policy and clinical practice.

HEV Indications in the Reproductive Tissues

The discovery that HEV is present in male reproductive organs is a crucial one in favor of the theory linking HEV infection to male infertility. Research has indicated that HEV is capable of infecting and replicating in the epididymis, semen, and testicular tissue.

Findings in Semen: HEV RNA was found in the semen of those who were infected, indicating that the virus may be excreted in seminal fluid. This discovery suggests that HEV may be sexually transmitted and may endure in the male reproductive system.

Testicular Infection: Evidence that the virus can infect and proliferate in male reproductive tissues has been further supported by the detection of HEV in the testes of infected humans and animals. This involvement of the testicles may interfere with regular spermatogenesis and hormone production, leading to infertility.

Observations in Clinical Practice

Additional proof that there is a connection between HEV and male infertility has come from clinical observations. Men with HEV infection have been shown to have lower sperm quality and quantity in case reports and small-scale research.

Sperm Quality: A number of studies have shown that men with HEV infection have different sperm quality. Reduced sperm concentration, aberrant sperm morphology, and decreased sperm motility are some of these alterations; these are all important factors to consider when evaluating male fertility.

Cases of Infertility: A few case studies have detailed men who experienced acute HEV infection and then became infertile. Despite being somewhat uncommon, these cases offer crucial information about the possible effects of HEV infection on reproduction.

Results of Ohio State University Research

Researchers at The Ohio State University have made significant discoveries that have illuminated the possible processes through which HEV may affect male fertility. Their research on animal models—pigs in particular—has yielded important information about how HEV affects and infects the male reproductive system

Design and Methodology of the Study

Using pigs as a model, the Ohio State University research team devised a series of experiments to examine the impact of HEV infection on male reproductive health. Pigs are a perfect model for researching reproductive health issues because of how similar their reproductive structure is to that of people.

HEV inoculation: To determine how the infection affected the male pigs' ability to reproduce, the researchers gave them a HEV injection and kept an eye on the animals for a few weeks. Periodically, blood, semen, and tissue samples were collected for analysis as part of the study.

Fluorescence Microscopy: The researchers investigated the presence of HEV particles in the semen and reproductive tissues of the infected pigs using sophisticated fluorescence microscopy techniques. This made it possible for the virus to be precisely localized within the reproductive system.

Important Results

The Ohio State University study's results have shed important light on the possible effects of HEV on the health of male reproduction. Among the main conclusions of their research are:

Viral Shedding in Semen: At least 19% of the sperm cells taken from the animals 84 days after inoculation had viral particles linked to them, indicating the presence of HEV in the semen of infected pigs, according to the researchers. This provides credence to the theories that HEV can be sexually transferred and that it can live for long stretches of time in the male reproductive system.

Sperm Quality and Structure: Examination of the sperm from infected pigs showed that the sperm cells had suffered severe harm, including changes to their structure and decreased motility. These alterations show compromised sperm function, which may be linked to infertility.

Viral particle infectivity: It was discovered that the HEV particles in the semen were contagious, able to infect and start the reproduction of human liver cells in culture. This indicates that the virus is still active and has the ability to infect new tissues and people.

Mechanisms of Infertility Caused by HEVs

For the purpose of creating methods that will effectively lessen the impact of HEV on male reproductive health, it is imperative to comprehend the mechanisms by which it causes infertility. The Ohio State University study, in conjunction with other research, has determined multiple plausible pathways via which HEV may hinder male fertility

Direct Infection with Virus

Direct harm to sperm cells and reproductive tissues is one of the main ways that HEV may result in infertility. Given that HEV is found in the testes and semen, it is likely that the virus can enter these tissues, multiply, and cause harm to cells as well as reduced function.

Testicular Inflammation: Orchitis, or inflammation of the testes, is a result of HEV infection. The sensitive testicular tissues involved in spermatogenesis—the process by which sperm are produced—may be harmed by this inflammation. The infection can cause the release of inflammatory cytokines, which can worsen tissue damage and impair normal testicular function.

Damage to Sperm Cells: Direct HEV infection of sperm cells can result in aberrant morphology and function. Reduced motility, changed morphology, and decreased viability are all possible in damaged sperm cells, and these characteristics are crucial for male fertility. It appears that HEV may obstruct the regular process of fertilization because virus particles are found on the heads of sperm cells.

Effects Mediated by Immunity

The onset of infertility may also be influenced by the immune system's reaction to a HEV infection. The immune system can harm host organs, including the reproductive system, even though it is necessary for eliminating viral infections.

Autoimmune Reactions: The immune system's erroneous attack on its own tissues might occasionally result from the immunological response to HEV. This may result in autoimmune orchitis, a disorder in which the testes are attacked by the immune system, inflaming them and harming the spermatogenic cells.

Prolonged Inflammation: The reproductive system may experience protracted inflammation as a result of a chronic HEV infection. Prolonged inflammatory reactions may cause the testicular tissue to fibrose, or scar, which will reduce its capacity to generate healthy sperm. Prolonged inflammation may additionally disrupt the hormonal balance necessary for normal reproductive function.

Effects Mediated by Immunity

The onset of infertility may also be influenced by the immune system's reaction to a HEV infection. The immune system can harm host organs, including the reproductive system, even though it is necessary for eliminating viral infections.

Autoimmune Reactions: The immune system's erroneous attack on its own tissues might occasionally result from the immunological response to HEV. This may result in autoimmune orchitis, a disorder in which the testes are attacked by the immune system, inflaming them and harming the spermatogenic cells.

Prolonged Inflammation: The reproductive system may experience protracted inflammation as a result of a chronic HEV infection. Prolonged inflammatory reactions may cause the testicular tissue to fibrose, or scar, which will reduce its capacity to generate healthy sperm. Prolonged inflammation may additionally disrupt the hormonal balance necessary for normal reproductive function.

Possible Long-Term Repercussions

There is growing worry that chronic HEV infection may have long-term repercussions on fertility, even though the long-term effects of HEV infection on male reproductive health are not fully understood.

Chronic HEV Infection: HEV infection can develop chronic in immunocompromised people and last for months or even years. Men who have a persistent HEV infection may experience long-term fertility problems as a result of the reproductive tissues being seriously damaged.

Secondary Complications: Long-term HEV-induced liver damage may potentially indirectly affect male fertility. The body's overall hormonal balance can be impacted by liver failure, which can change how hormones are metabolized and cleared from the body. Reproductive function may also be further hampered by the systemic symptoms of chronic liver disease, which include exhaustion and poor general health.

Consequences for Clinical Practice and Public Health

The possible association between male infertility and HEV has important ramifications for clinical and public health. A multimodal strategy including public education, diagnostic testing, and preventive measures is needed to address this problem.

Education and Public Awareness

It is essential to increase knowledge regarding the possible effects of HEV on male reproductive health in order to facilitate early detection and prevention. Particularly in areas where the virus is widespread, public health campaigns should emphasize informing the public about the dangers of contracting HEV infection.

Targeted Education: It is important to focus educational efforts on high-risk groups, such as those who live in unsanitary environments, consume undercooked or raw pork products, and men who work in jobs that expose them to animals frequently. These ads ought to provide information on the possible effects of HEV infection on reproduction.

Promotion of Safe Practices: To lower the risk of HEV infection, public health messages should stress the need of using safe food handling and cooking techniques. This entails making sure that meat, particularly hog products, is cooked throughly as well as providing clean water and sanitary facilities.

Diagnostic Evaluation and Inspection

Better diagnostic procedures and HEV infection screening can assist identify people who may have reproductive issues and direct the necessary course of treatment.

Semen Testing: Potential cases of HEV-induced infertility may be found by looking for HEV in semen samples from men in high-risk groups or with unexplained infertility. Regular fertility examinations could include a semen test for HEV RNA.

Comprehensive Testing: Widespread availability of comprehensive diagnostic testing for HEV, such as molecular testing for viral RNA and serological testing for antibodies, is necessary. This would make it easier to identify HEV infection early and start the right treatment right away.

Preventive Actions

Protecting male reproductive health requires taking preventative steps to lower the incidence of HEV infection. Vaccination, better hygiene, and focused interventions for high-risk populations are some of these strategies.

Vaccination: The incidence of HEV infection could be considerably decreased by the creation and implementation of a HEV vaccine. The HEV 239 vaccine is presently accessible in China, but more work needs to be done to make it available everywhere, especially in areas where HEV prevalence is high.

Sanitation and Hygiene: One of the most important ways to stop HEV epidemics is to provide access to clean water and sanitation facilities. Promoting good hygiene, improving water quality, and putting policies in place to lessen HEV pollution in the environment should be the main goals of public health campaigns.

focused Interventions: People in high-risk vocations that include a lot of animal contact or those who live in areas where HEV outbreaks happen frequently ought to seek focused interventions. This might involve immunization, routine screening, and instruction on safe conduct.

The growing body of research demonstrates a serious and little-known public health concern: the association between male infertility and the Hepatitis E Virus (HEV). Important insights into the possible pathways by which HEV can affect male reproductive health—including direct viral harm, immune-mediated effects, and hormonal disruptions—have been gained from research undertaken by The Ohio State University and other investigations. Comprehending these pathways is crucial in formulating efficacious approaches to alleviate the influence of HEV on male fertility.

This connection has broad ramifications for professional practice, public health policy, and personal wellbeing. To address this issue, it is imperative to undertake preventative measures, improve diagnostic testing and screening, and raise public awareness. Translating research findings into practical public health interventions is crucial to safeguard and enhance men's reproductive health globally, especially as investigations into the full extent of HEV's influence on reproductive health continue.

Chapter 5

Hydrogen Evolution in Sperm and Semen

HEV Is Present on Sperm Cell Heads

A shocking finding from recent studies is that sperm cells have the Hepatitis E Virus (HEV) on their heads. This discovery raises concerns regarding the possible sexual transmission of HEV and its effects on reproductive health, with consequences for both human and animal fertility.

Understanding via Fluorescence Microscopy

One effective method for researching viral infections at the cellular level is fluorescence microscopy. Viral particles can be marked with fluorescent markers, which allows researchers to precisely examine how the particles interact with host cells and tissues.

HEV detection: HEV particles connected to sperm cell heads have been found by researchers using fluorescence microscopy. The presence and possible influence of these viral particles on sperm function are shown by the bright fluorescent spots that emerge on the sperm surface.

Localization investigations: In-depth localization investigations have demonstrated that HEV attaches and enters the host cell more easily by selectively binding to particular receptors on the surface of sperm cells. The effectiveness of viral infection and replication within the male reproductive system may be improved by this targeted binding.

Consequences for Human Reproduction

Concerns over HEV's possible impact on human fertility have been raised since it was found on sperm cells. Because sperm cells are essential to fertilization, any changes to their composition or functionality may have an adverse effect on male fertility and the quality of offspring.

Effect on the Quality of Sperm

Sperm cell HEV infection may have a significant impact on the motility, morphology, and viability of the sperm. According to studies, viruses can change the sperm's biochemical makeup, which can impact the sperm's ability to travel and penetrate the egg during fertilization.

Reduced motility: Sperm cells damaged by HEV may have less motility, which will make it more difficult for them to pass through the female reproductive system and get to the egg. Male infertility is frequently caused by decreased sperm motility, which can drastically lower the likelihood of pregnancy.

Abnormal Morphology: Sperm cell malformations, such as malformed heads or tails, can also result from HEV infection. Fertility may be further compromised by these anomalies because they may hinder the sperm's ability to attach to and penetrate the egg.

Reduced Viability: Research has indicated that sperm cell viability may be impacted by HEV infection, making it impossible for the cells to fertilize an egg. Male fertility can be severely hampered by reduced sperm viability, which also raises the possibility of infertility.

Possibility of Transmission to Children

Concerns over the virus's possible transfer to offspring during conception are raised by the discovery of HEV on sperm cells. Congenital HEV infection may result from the virus infecting the developing embryo if viral particles are still adhered to sperm cells after fertilization.

Vertical Transmission: Serious effects for fetal development could result from the vertical transmission of HEV from father to offspring through infected sperm cells. Fetal discomfort, intrauterine growth restriction, and stillbirth have all been linked to HEV infection during pregnancy, underscoring the possible dangers of congenital HEV infection.

Effect on Embryonic Development: Normal fetal development may be disrupted by HEV infection in the early phases of embryonic development, which could result in congenital defects or developmental disorders. More research is necessary to properly understand the long-term implications of prenatal HEV infection on the health and well-being of offspring.

Consequences for Animal Reproduction

HEV infection of sperm cells affects not just human fertility but also animal reproduction, especially in farm species like pigs. HEV is mostly found in pigs, and spreading the virus through contaminated semen could have serious repercussions for animal production and breeding initiatives.

Effects on the Reproduction of Swine

Swine reproductive and productivity may be jeopardized if boars, the male breeding pigs employed in artificial insemination systems, contract HEV infection. The profitability of swine operations may eventually be impacted by lower fertility and conception rates in sows due to the presence of HEV on sperm cells.

Decreased Sow Fertility: HEV-infected semen can cause a sow to become less fertile and more likely to have reproductive failure. Damage from HEVs to sperm cells may hinder their capacity to fertilize eggs, which could lead to smaller litter sizes and decreased output in general.

Transmission to Offspring: The infection cycle in swine herds may be sustained by the transfer of HEV from boars to piglets via contaminated semen. Piglets with congenital HEV infection may experience delayed growth, higher mortality, and other health issues, which would further reduce the profitability of swine production.

Techniques of Management

Swine producers may need to use targeted management methods and biosecurity measures to lessen the effect of HEV on animal reproduction.

Semen Screening: By routinely checking boar semen for HEV, it may be possible to detect sick animals and stop the virus from spreading through artificial insemination. To guarantee the quality and security of semen used for insemination, standard breeding procedures should include semen testing for HEV RNA utilizing molecular diagnostic tools.

Programs for Vaccination: Vaccinating boars against HEV may add another line of defense against the spread of the virus and the loss of reproductive potential. Lower virus levels in the semen produced by vaccinated boars may lessen the chance of HEV transmission to sows and their progeny.

Biosecurity Measures: To stop the introduction and spread of HEV among swine herds, stringent biosecurity measures such as quarantine guidelines and semen sanitation practices should be put in place. In breeding facilities and boar studs, the danger of virus contamination can be reduced with the use of appropriate sanitation protocols and hygiene standards.

Fertility in humans and animals is significantly impacted by the presence of HEV on sperm cells. HEV infection of sperm cells may reduce sperm quality and raise the risk of infertility in humans, but it may also affect swine productivity and reproduction in animals. Concerns regarding vertical transmission to progeny and its effect on fetal development are raised by the possible spread of HEV through contaminated semen. Developing focused ways to lessen the impact of the virus on fertility in both humans and animals is crucial as research into the complexity of HEV infection and its impacts on reproductive health continues. Through comprehending the processes behind HEV-caused infertility and putting suitable control measures in place, we can protect people's reproductive health and guarantee the sustainability of of livestock production systems.

SECTION III:

The Swine Industry's Use of HEVs

Chapter 6

Pig HEV Infection

Pig infections with the hepatitis E virus (HEV) have become a major concern in the swine business, with implications for food safety and animal health. HEV is mostly stored in pigs, and spreading the virus throughout swine herds can result in financial losses as well as threats to the general public's health. Comprehending the intricacies of HEV infection in swine is crucial in order to formulate efficacious measures for mitigation and to preserve the authenticity of the pork supply chain.

Using Pigs as a Model to Examine HEV

Since pigs are a natural host for HEV, they are a valuable model animal to study the biology, pathology, and transmission of the virus. Pigs are an appropriate model organism for HEV due to a number of reasons.

Analytical and Physiological Similarities: Pigs are a great model for researching HEV infection in relation to reproductive health since their anatomy and physiology are quite similar to human reproductive systems. Pigs can contract HEV just like humans can, and they can shed the virus in their semen, which makes it easier to examine how the infection spreads through sexual activity.

Ease of Husbandry: Researchers can conduct controlled studies to explore various aspects of HEV infection in pigs since they are relatively straightforward to handle and maintain in laboratory settings. Research is made easier by the availability of specific-pathogen-free (SPF) pig colonies, which provide pigs immune from other infectious organisms that could skew study results.

Similar Disease Course: Comparable Disease Course: The clinical signs of HEV infection in pigs, such as acute hepatitis and fecal viral shedding, are quite similar to those seen in humans. Researching HEV infection in pigs can reveal important information on the processes involved in viral replication, host immunological responses, and the development of animal and human diseases.

Research on Immunization and Results

Studies involving experimental inoculation have been crucial in clarifying the dynamics of HEV infection in pigs and the consequences it poses for the health of swine. In these research, pigs are given HEV infection under controlled circumstances, and the animals are then observed for histological alterations, clinical symptoms, and viral shedding.

Inoculation Procedures: To replicate the natural methods of infection, pigs are normally infected with HEV orally or intravenously. Purified viral particles, infectious cell culture supernatants, or fecal samples from animals infected with HEV can all be used as the inoculum. Pig control groups are frequently included in studies to compare the effects of infection with those of non-infected animals.

Clinical Manifestations: Inoculated pigs may experience symptoms similar to those of acute HEV infection in humans, such as jaundice, lethargy, and anorexia. However, a large number of infected pigs show either moderate clinical indications or remain asymptomatic, underscoring the variation in illness presentation.

Viral Shedding: Pigs infected with HEV excrete the virus, which can contaminate the environment and spread to other animals. Viral RNA in fecal samples is found and measured using quantitative PCR techniques, which enables researchers to track the dynamics of viral shedding over time.

Histological abnormalities: Hepatocellular necrosis, inflammation, and fibrosis are among the typical histological abnormalities in the liver that are frequently found during post-mortem examinations of infected pigs. These alterations offer information about the etiology of HEV infection in pigs and are suggestive of acute hepatitis.

The high frequency of asymptomatic cases—in which infected animals exhibit no outward symptoms of illness—is one of the noteworthy characteristics of HEV infection in pigs. Because asymptomatic infections might cause an animal to unintentionally shed the virus and become a source of transmission for other pigs and possibly people, they present challenges for disease surveillance and control efforts.

Subclinical Infections: A significant percentage of pigs infected with HEV infections do not exhibit overt symptoms of sickness, making subclinical or silent infections common. These animals may show slight histological alterations in the liver or temporary increases in liver enzymes, but they generally maintain clinical health.

Viral Shedding: Asymptomatic pigs can nevertheless excrete HEV at levels similar to those of symptomatic animals, even in the absence of any clinical symptoms. This puts humans who come into contact with diseased animals or their excrement at danger of environmental contamination, as well as transmission to other pigs in the same herd.

Chronic Shedding: Some pigs may develop into chronic HEV shedders, releasing the virus into their feces on a regular basis for a considerable amount of time. In addition to potentially extending the virus's survival in the environment, chronic shedders are crucial to the upkeep of HEV circulation in swine herds.

For the swine business, HEV infection in pigs poses a complicated and multidimensional dilemma with ramifications for public health, food safety, and animal health. HEV is naturally found in pigs, and swine herd transmission of the virus can result in financial losses as well as health hazards to humans via zoonotic transmission pathways. Studies on experimental inoculation have yielded important insights into the dynamics of HEV infection in pigs, including the disease's histological abnormalities, clinical signs, and viral shedding patterns. The high incidence of asymptomatic cases in pigs makes it difficult to monitor the disease and manage it; better diagnostic techniques and focused interventions are therefore required to lower the spread of HEV throughout swine herds. Through learning more about HEV infection in pigs and its implications for swine health and food safety, we can develop effective strategies to mitigate the impact of the virus on both animal and human populations.

Chapter 7

HEV and Artificial Insemination

In the swine business, artificial insemination (AI) is a popular reproductive technique that facilitates the productive generation of pig litters and the genetic enhancement of animal populations. However, questions concerning the security of AI procedures and the possibility of viral transmission through donor sperm have been raised in light of the discovery of the Hepatitis E Virus (HEV) as a possible threat to swine health and reproduction. This chapter presents an overview of artificial intelligence (AI) in the swine business, investigates the possibility of HEV transmission through donor sperm, and talks about industry procedures and risk management issues.

Synopsis of Artificial Insemination in the Pork Sector

A reproductive method called artificial insemination is used to impregnate female animals in the absence of natural mating. AI is frequently used in the swine business to breed sows with superior boar semen, producing more controlled and predictable breeding results. Boars' semen is collected, its quality assessed, and sows are inseminated at the best period for pregnancy.

Advantages of Artificial Fertilization

Genetic Improvement: AI enables pig farmers to carefully choose sows that possess high-performance characteristics, like quick growth rates, effective feed conversion, and resistance to disease. Producers can quicken the pace of genetic advancement in their herds by utilizing the semen of excellent boars with desired genetic traits.

Disease Control: During natural mating, AI helps lower the chance of sexually transmitted infections (STIs) and other reproductive illnesses spreading between animals. Pig farmers can reduce the entrance and spread of infections within their herds and enhance the general health of their herds by testing and screening boars for infectious agents.

Efficiency and Productivity: By improving breeding schedules and reducing the amount of time between pregnancies, AI helps farmers to maximize the reproductive potential of their breeding animals. Producers are able to boost the number of piglets born per litter and increase overall operational efficiency by inseminating multiple sows with a single ejaculate from a boar.

Important AI Process Steps

Semen collecting: A sophisticated artificial vagina or collecting device is used to harvest semen from boars. The quality and fertility of the semen are then determined by analyzing its volume, concentration, motility, and morphology.

Semen Processing: To increase the duration and fertilizing potential of semen, it is processed to eliminate seminal plasma and debris, concentrate sperm cells, and lengthen the semen with an appropriate diluent.

Insemination: Using a catheter or insemination pistol, processed semen is put into insemination doses and inseminated into the reproductive tract of female pigs (sows or gilts). To guarantee the best possible conception rates and litter sizes, timing of insemination is essential.

Possibility of Transmitting HEV via Donor Sperm

Concerns over the security of AI procedures and the possibility of viral transmission through donor sperm have been raised by the discovery of HEV as a possible threat to swine reproduction. HEV can spread by fecal-oral pathways, such as tainted semen, and is excreted by sick animals. Numerous investigations have reported the presence of HEV in boar semen, underscoring the possibility of viral transmission via AI procedures.

Research Results

Semen Detection: Research has shown that HEV RNA is present in boar semen, suggesting that the virus is present in the reproductive tissues of infected animals. The virus's ability to stick to sperm cells' heads has been discovered, which raises questions about how it may infect female pigs during AI treatments.

Infectivity in Culture: Experimental research has shown that the herpesvirus (HEV) particles found in swine semen are contagious and able to multiply in cultured cells. This implies that the virus is still active and able to infect vulnerable hosts, such as female pigs injected with tainted semen.

Transmission to Offspring: In certain instances, vertical transmission of HEV from boars to piglets has been reported, suggesting that the virus can be transferred from parent to child via contaminated semen. The possibility of congenital HEV infection in piglets born to infected sows inseminated with tainted semen is raised by this

Hazard Contributors

Asymptomatic Shedding: A large number of boars infected with HEV may shed the virus asymptomatically in their semen without exhibiting any outward symptoms of sickness.

Disease detection and control are made more difficult by asymptomatic shedding, since sick animals may remain undetected and continue to disseminate the virus among swine herds.

Herd Prevalence: Variations in geography can be observed in the prevalence of HEV infection in swine herds, which can be impacted by various factors including the size of the herd, management strategies, and biosecurity protocols. Exposure to HEV-contaminated semen and the risk of viral transmission through AI techniques are both increased in high herd prevalence situations.

Industry Customs and Difficulties

In order to manage the danger of HEV transmission through AI methods and ensure donor sperm safety, swine farmers must overcome a number of obstacles. Industry norms and difficulties consist of:

Screening and Testing: To reduce the risk of viral transmission, screening and testing procedures for HEV infection in boars and donor semen must be put into place. Accurate illness identification, however, may face difficulties due to the low sensitivity of existing HEV diagnostic assays in identifying low quantities of viral RNA in semen.

Biosecurity Measures: Using AI techniques, improving biosecurity measures in swine herds and boar studs can help lower the risk of HEV transmission. This entails putting stringent cleanliness procedures into place, separating contaminated animals, and keeping boars away from possible sources of infection.

Vaccination Programs: The creation and application of HEV vaccinations for swine may offer an extra instrument for managing viral spread and safeguarding the well-being of animals. The effectiveness of currently available vaccinations in lowering viral shedding and decreasing disease transmission, however, has not yet been thoroughly assessed. Vaccine development is still underway.

Regulatory Oversight: In order to monitor AI processes and guarantee adherence to industry norms and regulations, regulatory bodies are essential. Standardizing procedures and reducing the chance of viral transmission through donor sperm can be achieved by establishing explicit regulatory frameworks for HEV testing and management in swine studs and AI institutes.

In the swine business, artificial insemination is essential for effective breeding plans and genetic population enhancement. However, questions concerning the security of AI procedures and the possibility of viral transmission through donor sperm have been raised in light of the discovery of the Hepatitis E Virus (HEV) as a possible threat to swine health and reproduction. The identification of diseased animals, the application of biosecurity precautions, and regulatory monitoring of AI procedures are among the difficulties faced by swine producers in controlling the risk of HEV spread. Producers can protect the integrity of the pork supply chain and reduce the risk of HEV transmission through AI procedures by addressing these issues and putting in place the necessary control measures.

Chapter 8

Consequences for the Economy and Health

The endemicity of the hepatitis E virus (HEV) in swine populations has serious health and economic consequences for both the swine industry and the general public's health. The frequency of HEV in swine populations, its effects on the health and productivity of swine reproduction, and the cost-benefit analysis of HEV screening and immunization programs are all covered in this chapter.

HEV Endemicity in Populations of Swine

HEV is endemic in swine populations all throughout the world, and different geographical areas and production practices have varied prevalence rates. HEV naturally occurs in swine, and fecal samples from both healthy and sick pigs frequently include the virus. HEV endemicity in swine populations is caused by a number of factors, including:

High Shedding Rates: Pigs with the infection may excrete large amounts of HEV in their feces, which can contaminate the environment and spread throughout swine herds. The age, sex, and immunological status of the animals are some of the variables that can affect the rate of HEV shedding.

Horizontal Transmission: Pigs can contract HEV from one another by fecal-oral routes, which include consuming contaminated feed, water, or environmental surfaces, as well as direct contact with diseased animals. Inadequate hygiene and overcrowding in housing can make HEV transmission in swine herds worse.

Vertical Transmission: During pregnancy or lactation, sows can transmit HEV vertically to piglets, which might result in congenital infection in the young animals. The gestational stage, mother antibodies, and other factors can all affect the prevalence of vertical transmission.

Influence on Swine Productivity and Reproductive Health

Swine HEV infection can have serious effects on reproductive health and production, which can impact litter sizes, breeding success, and herd performance as a whole. The following are some effects of HEV on swine reproductive health:

Decreased Fertility: Lower conception rates and decreased fertility rates in boars and sows might result in miscarried or delayed pregnancies. Reproductive tissue viral replication has the potential to reduce gamete quality and fertilization potential, which could result in less than ideal breeding outcomes.

Abortion and Stillbirth: Pregnant sows who are infected with HEV have an increased chance of abortion, stillbirth, and neonatal mortality. Placental insufficiency, intrauterine growth restriction, and infection-associated fetal distress can all lead to unfavorable pregnancy outcomes and financial losses for swine farmers.

Inadequate Growth: Congenital HEV infection in pigs can cause poor growth, which can lower weight gain, raise mortality, and lower production all around. Long-term financial losses for swine producers could be the consequence of chronic infection and recurrent HEV shedding in piglets.

Cost-Benefit Evaluation of Vaccination and Screening Programs for HEVs

In order to lessen the influence of the virus on swine health and production, control techniques including screening and vaccination programs are becoming more and more popular, given the negative effects HEV endemicity has on swine populations' health and economy. Evaluating the possible costs and advantages of putting HEV screening and vaccination programs into place is the task of a cost-benefit analysis.

Programs for Screening

Cost of Testing: Sample collection, laboratory testing, and data analysis are among the costs associated with screening swine herds for HEV infection. The cost of diagnostic tests, such as serological or PCR assays, varies according to the quantity and frequency of samples tested.

Benefits of Early Detection: The benefits of early detection include the ability to identify sick animals, carry out focused control actions, and stop the virus from spreading throughout swine herds. Early identification of HEV infection is achieved by screening programs. Prompt intervention has the potential to decrease the prevalence of reproductive problems, boost breeding results, and improve the general health and productivity of herds.

Cost of Disease Outbreaks: The financial consequences of HEV outbreaks in swine herds include expenses for lower productivity, higher mortality rates, and decreased fertility. outbreaks of disease may result in losses due to aborted litters, neonatal mortality, and reduced market value of affected animals.

Immunization Schedules

Cost of Vaccine Development: The price of conducting clinical studies, obtaining regulatory permission, manufacturing, and research and development are all included in the cost of creating and licensing HEV vaccines for swine. The creation of vaccines may necessitate a substantial time and resource commitment in order to guarantee safety, effectiveness, and industrial scalability.

Benefits of Vaccination: Vaccinating pigs against HEV can minimize viral shedding, stop disease transmission within swine herds, and offer long-term protection against viral infection. Pig farmers may profit more from vaccinated animals due to better reproductive outcomes, lower death rates, and higher growth performance.

Cost-Effectiveness Analysis: In this analysis, the costs and benefits of vaccination programs are compared to those of other control measures or to no intervention at all. When assessing the cost-effectiveness of vaccination regimens, variables such vaccine cost per dose, duration of immunity, and efficacy are taken into account.

The endemicity of the hepatitis E virus (HEV) in swine populations has important health and economic ramifications for both the swine industry and the general public. HEV infection can have an adverse effect on the reproductive health and production of pigs, resulting in lower fertility, higher rates of abortion, and poor growth outcomes for piglets. Mitigating the impact of HEV on swine productivity and health can be achieved by the use of control measures including vaccination and screening programs. Evaluating the possible costs and advantages of screening and vaccination programs in relation to the financial losses brought on by HEV outbreaks in swine herds is the process of doing a cost-benefit analysis of HEV control methods. Pork farmers may safeguard the wellbeing and health of their animals as well as the long-term viability of their businesses by making investments in proactive disease prevention and control techniques.

SECTION IV

Wider Consequences of HEV

Chapter 9

Neurological and Pancreatic Illnesses

Historically recognized for its effects on liver function, hepatitis E virus (HEV) infection has been linked more and more to a variety of extrahepatic symptoms, such as neurological and pancreatic conditions. Through a combination of clinical observations and experimental investigations, this chapter explores the growing body of data that links HEV to neurological problems and pancreatic abnormalities.

Adjacent Pancreatic Disorders with HEVs

Evidence indicates that HEV can impact pancreatic function and play a role in the development of pancreatic diseases, despite its primary target being the liver. The connection between HEV infection and pancreatic disorders has been investigated in a number of clinical and experimental investigations, such as:

Acute Pancreatitis: This condition is marked by inflammation of the pancreas and can cause excruciating pain in the abdomen as well as nausea and vomiting. Research has documented instances of acute HEV infection linked to acute pancreatitis, indicating a possible pathogenic relationship between the virus and inflammation of the pancreas.

Chronic Pancreatitis: Chronic pancreatitis is a chronic inflammatory disease that can cause irreversible harm to the pancreas as well as decreased function. Chronic HEV infection has been suggested as a potential initiator of chronic pancreatitis, while the underlying processes of this correlation remain unclear.

Autoimmune Pancreatitis: An autoimmune-mediated inflammation of the pancreas is the hallmark of this type of chronic pancreatitis. According to newly available data, HEV infection may cause autoimmune reactions in people who are vulnerable, which could result in the development of autoimmune pancreatitis and other autoimmune diseases.

Evidence from Clinical and Experimental Research

Epidemiological Studies: Compared to healthy controls, individuals with acute and chronic pancreatitis had higher rates of HEV infection. These findings raise the possibility that HEV and pancreatic illnesses are related. To prove that HEV infection and pancreatic disorders are causally related, more investigation is necessary.

Animal Models: Research employing HEV-infected animal models has shed light on the pathophysiology of diseases of the pancreas linked to HEV infection. These investigations have shown that the HEV virus plays a role in the development of pancreatic disorders by demonstrating viral replication in pancreatic tissues, inducing pancreatic inflammation, and disrupting pancreatic function after infection.

Neurological Issues Associated with HEV

Apart from its impact on the liver and pancreas, HEV infection has been connected to several neurological issues, such as:

GBS, or Guillain-Barré Syndrome, is an uncommon neurological condition.

characterized by paralysis, numbness, and weakness of the muscles; frequently occurs after an acute infection. Numerous investigations have revealed a link between HEV infection and GBS, indicating that the virus may cause autoimmune-mediated nerve injury in those who are vulnerable.

Neurological Symptoms: Meningitis, peripheral neuropathy, encephalitis, and other neurological symptoms have all been linked to HEV infection. These neurological issues could be brought on by a HEV infection that triggers immune-mediated processes or by a direct viral invasion of the brain system.

Chronic Neurological Sequelae: Cognitive decline, motor dysfunction, and sensory abnormalities are examples of chronic neurological sequelae that some patients with HEV-associated neurological problems may encounter. The quality of life and morbidity of the patient may be significantly impacted by these long-term consequences.

Evidence from Clinical and Experimental Research

Case Studies: Clinical case studies have shown that patients with both acute and chronic HEV infection might experience neurological problems, indicating that the virus may have neurotropic potential. Acute hepatitis may be followed by or concomitant with neurological symptoms, which emphasizes the necessity for healthcare professionals to be more knowledgeable about HEV-associated neurological problems.

Pathophysiological Mechanisms: The pathophysiological mechanisms behind HEV-induced neurological problems have been clarified by experimental research employing in vitro cell culture systems and animal models. These investigations have shed light on the intricate interactions between the virus and the neurological system by showing viral multiplication in neural cells, neuroinflammatoryreactions, and disruption of the blood-brain barrier integrity after HEV infection.

Recognizing the wider ramifications of HEV infection beyond liver disease is crucial, as evidence is mounting that links the Hepatitis E Virus (HEV) to neurological and pancreatic problems. The possible correlation between HEV and pancreatic illnesses, such as acute, chronic, and autoimmune pancreatitis, has been illuminated by both clinical observations and experimental investigations. HEV infection has also been linked to encephalitis, peripheral neuropathy, and Guillain-Barré Syndrome (GBS), among other neurological consequences, demonstrating the virus's neurotropic potential.

To determine the causal link between HEV infection and these extrahepatic symptoms, as well as to clarify the pathophysiological mechanisms underpinning pancreatic and neurological diseases linked with HEV infection, more research is required. Healthcare professionals must have a greater understanding of the wider clinical spectrum of HEV infection in order to identify and treat pancreatic and neurological problems in patients with HEV-associated liver disease in a timely manner. To lessen the burden of extrahepatic symptoms in HEV-infected persons, we can create targeted treatment strategies and enhance patient care by comprehending the complex nature of HEV infection and its effects on different organ systems.

Chapter 10

Policies and Public Health

Globally, the hepatitis E virus (HEV) presents serious public health risks that call for extensive preventive and control measures to lessen the virus's negative effects on human health. The present approaches to preventing and controlling HEV transmission and the associated illness burden are examined in this chapter, along with suggestions for public health interventions and policy implications.

Current Approaches to HEV Control and Prevention
Better Hygiene and Sanitation

In order to stop the fecal-oral transmission of HEV, it is essential to promote access to clean water and sanitation facilities.

Public health programs that highlight safe food handling techniques, good hand hygiene, and sanitation measures can help lower the community's risk of contracting HEV infection.

Improved Monitoring and Identification

For early identification and response, surveillance systems that track illness trends, identify outbreak clusters, and monitor HEV prevalence must be strengthened.

Timely diagnosis and effective patient care can be facilitated by developing sensitive and specific laboratory tests that improve diagnostic capabilities for HEV infection.

Immunization Schedules

One approach that shows promise for avoiding infection and lowering disease burden is the development and distribution of HEV vaccinations.

Immunization of high-risk groups, such as those with chronic liver disease and pregnant women, can help shield these populations from serious consequences from HEV infection.

Blood Safety Procedures

Ensuring blood safety requires putting in place screening procedures and donor selection standards to reduce the possibility of HEV infection through organ transplantation and blood transfusions.

Screening blood donations for HEV RNA or antibodies using serological assays or nucleic acid testing (NAT) can assist in identifying and excluding possibly infectious donors.

Regulations Concerning Food Safety

Lowering the risk of foodborne transmission depends on enforcing food safety laws and standards to avoid HEV contamination of food products, especially pig and shellfish.

By putting into practice techniques like pasteurization, cooking, and careful handling of raw meat and shellfish, HEV can be inactivated and consumer exposure can be reduced.

Suggestions for Public Health Measures
Campaigns for Health Education and Awareness

People can be empowered to protect themselves from infection by initiating public health education campaigns to increase knowledge about HEV transmission channels, risk factors, and preventative actions.

The efficacy of health education programs can be increased by involving legislators, community leaders, and healthcare professionals in the dissemination of correct information and the encouragement of preventative practices.

Interventions Based in the Community

Increasing community involvement in HEV preventive and control initiatives and organizing available resources can help improve the ability of the local community to deal with the disease load.

Health outcomes can be enhanced by putting into practice community-based interventions that are suited to the particular requirements and preferences of target communities, such as immunization drives, screening programs, and sanitation initiatives.

Cooperation Across Sectors

To create integrated strategies for HEV control, encourage cooperation and coordination between public health organizations, medical professionals, veterinary services, food safety authorities, and other pertinent stakeholders.

Encouraging multidisciplinary research and knowledge sharing amongst fields like immunology, virology, epidemiology, and environmental health can help to clarify the dynamics of HEV transmission holistically and guide evidence-based responses.

Future Directions and Policy Implications
Policy Formulation and Execution

Developing evidence-based policies and standards for HEV diagnosis, treatment, and prevention is crucial to directing public health practice and guaranteeing uniformity in methodology among various authorities.

Prioritizing resources and fostering political commitment to addressing the HEV burden can be achieved by including HEV control strategies into national infectious disease control programs and public health agendas.

Innovation and Research

Innovative preventive and control measures can be developed by funding research and innovation to increase our knowledge of HEV pathophysiology, immunology, and epidemiology.

Encouraging research endeavors focused on creating novel diagnostic tools, vaccines, antiviral treatments, and vector management strategies can expedite the attainment of HEV eradication objectives.

International Cooperation and Protest

In order to generate support for coordinated action and increase awareness of HEV as a global health issue, international cooperation and advocacy efforts should be strengthened.

collaborating with international organizations to create global strategies, exchange best practices, and standardize HEV control standards, such as the Food and Agriculture Organization (FAO) and the World Health Organization (WHO).

Globally, HEV poses a serious threat to public health and calls for coordinated action to stop the virus's spread and lessen its burden. The current approaches to prevention and control concentrate on boosting food safety, guaranteeing blood safety, establishing immunization programs, and increasing sanitation and surveillance. To address the complex nature of HEV transmission and disease, however, more funding is required for health education, community-based treatments, interdisciplinary research, and policy reform. Policymakers, healthcare professionals, and communities may collaborate to reduce the harm that high-energy vehicles (HEVs) cause to human health and to accomplish the worldwide objective of HEV elimination by implementing a comprehensive and integrated approach to HEV control.

Chapter 11

Research on HEVs and Their Prospects

Although research on the Hepatitis E virus (HEV) has advanced recently, there are still many unanswered questions about the epidemiology, pathophysiology, and clinical implications of the virus. This chapter examines the state of HEV research today, points out knowledge gaps, talks about new developments in HEV research, and suggests areas for future investigation that could lead to significant discoveries.

Research Gaps in Current HEVs
First, epidemiology

Insufficient knowledge about the prevalence, worldwide distribution, and dynamics of HEV transmission, especially in environments with limited resources and among vulnerable populations.

Inadequate understanding of how environmental variables, zoonotic transmission routes, and animal reservoirs affect the dynamics of HEV transmission.

Pathophysiology

Uncertainty about the immune escape tactics used by the virus, its persistence, and the mechanisms underpinning HEV replication.

Inadequate description of the relationships between the host and the virus, including innate immunity, cellular receptors, and viral tropism in various organ systems.

Clinical Signs and Symptoms

The clinical range of HEV infection, which includes asymptomatic instances, acute hepatitis, chronic infection, and extrahepatic symptoms, is not well understood.

Inadequate understanding of the risk factors, prognostic markers, and long-term consequences linked to neurological problems, pregnancy issues, and liver illness linked to HEV.

Diagnoses

For HEV detection, quantification, and genotyping, there are no defined diagnostic tests or methods, which causes variation in test performance and interpretation.

difficulties in obtaining trustworthy and reasonably priced diagnostic instruments in environments with limited resources, which impedes precise disease monitoring and patient care.

New Developments in HEV Research: Trends and Technologies
NGS, or Next-Generation Sequencing

NGS technologies enable thorough genomic analysis and molecular epidemiological research by providing hitherto unattainable insights into HEV diversity, evolution, and host adaptation.

Metagenomic and whole-genome sequencing techniques make it easier to find new HEV strains, virulence-causing genes, and possible therapeutic targets.

The Study of Systems Biology

Proteomics, metabolomics, transcriptomics, and genomes data are integrated by systems biology techniques to clarify the intricate host-pathogen dynamics and molecular processes involved in HEV infection

Pathogenesis of HEV, immunological responses, and disease development can be understood at the systems level through the use of network-based analysis and computational modeling tools.

Model Animals

creation of reliable animal models for the study of HEV infection, transmission, and pathogenesis, including as zebrafish, genetically engineered mice, and non-human primates.

Preclinical testing, mechanistic investigations, and controlled experimentation with antiviral medications and vaccine candidates for HEV are made possible by in vivo models.

Vaccinology and Immunology

improvements in immunological methods for analyzing host immune reactions to HEV infection, including single-cell sequencing, multiparameter flow cytometry, and epitope mapping.

Reverse vaccinology, structure-based antigen design, and adjuvant modification are used in the rational design of HEV vaccines to improve vaccine durability and efficacy.

Priorities for Upcoming Research and Possible Breakthroughs

Comprehending Transmission Dynamic

examining how host variables, foodborne transmission pathways, and environmental reservoirs affect the dynamics of HEV transmission in various epidemiological contexts.

combining multidisciplinary methods from the social sciences, ecology, and epidemiology to create risk assessment instruments and prediction models for the spread of HEVs.

Clarifying the Mechanisms of Pathogenesis:

utilizing sophisticated molecular virology and cell biology tools to decipher the molecular mechanisms of host-virus interactions, virulence factors, and HEV replication

determining genetic factors that influence the severity of the disease, host susceptibility factors, and biomarkers that can be used to forecast treatment outcomes and clinical outcomes.

Creating Innovative Interventions:

increasing the number of antiviral medications that target HEV entrance, replication, and assembly by using structure-based drug design, high-throughput screening, and drug repurposing.

optimizing adjuvant formulations, vaccine candidates, and immunization techniques to provide at-risk people with a strong and long-lasting protective immunity against HEV infection.

Converging Science and Application

converting research results for HEV prevention, diagnosis, and management into clinical guidelines, evidence-based public health actions, and policy recommendations.

bolstering international partnerships, capacity-building programs, and knowledge-sharing networks to hasten the conversion of scientific findings into observable health benefits.

Recent developments in immunology, computational sciences, and molecular biology have propelled HEV research to impressive new heights. Our knowledge of the epidemiology, pathophysiology, and clinical symptoms of HEV is still lacking in many areas. NGS, systems biology, animal models, immunology, and other emerging trends and technologies show promise in filling in these knowledge gaps and providing fresh perspectives on the biology and pathology of HEVs. The scientific community can lead the way for revolutionary discoveries in HEV research and public health practice by emphasizing research efforts, encouraging interdisciplinary collaboration, and utilizing creative approaches. This will eventually lessen the burden of HEV-related morbidity and mortality on a global scale.

In summary

The Hepatitis E Virus (HEV) poses intricate problems at the nexus of economic sustainability, animal welfare, and human health. We have examined the epidemiology, dynamics of transmission, clinical symptoms, and wider implications for reproductive health and the swine industry throughout this book to better understand the complex nature of HEV. Let's take a moment to review the most important conclusions and revelations from our investigation of HEV and discuss what this means for future studies, regulations, and business initiatives.

Key Findings and Insights Synopsis

HEV Epidemiology: HEV is distributed worldwide and can spread through a variety of channels, such as fecal-oral, zoonotic, and possibly sexual means. Effective disease control and prevention depend on an understanding of the intricate interactions between animal and human reservoirs.

Clinical Implications: Acute hepatitis, chronic infection, and extrahepatic consequences are only a few of the clinical symptoms that might result from HEV infection. Asymptomatic instances are also possible. Patients with impaired immune systems, those with underlying liver disease, and expectant mothers are most susceptible to negative consequences.

Reproductive Health: Due to its potential effects on male infertility and pregnancy outcomes, HEV has become a major reproductive health concern. Empirical evidence points to a possible connection between HEV infection and unfavorable pregnancy outcomes, as well as changes in sperm quality and fertility.

Impact of the Swine Industry: As a natural reservoir for the virus, the swine industry is essential to the dynamics of HEV transmission. Pigs with HEV infection frequently show no symptoms, but it can affect artificial insemination procedures, reproductive success, and herd productivity as a whole.

Last Words on the Impact of HEVs

Beyond just liver illness, HEVs have an impact on agricultural systems and reproductive health throughout the world. In order to effectively address the HEV burden, interdisciplinary collaboration, creative ideas, and evidence-based interventions are required, as demonstrated by the convergence of human and animal health. In order to effectively tackle this new threat, it is critical that we understand how public health, veterinary care, and food safety are intertwined as we negotiate the complexity of HEV.

Urge to Take Action
Researchers: To improve our knowledge of HEV epidemiology, pathophysiology, and transmission dynamics, fund cooperative research projects. Utilize cutting-edge technologies and multidisciplinary methods to create innovative therapies, monitoring techniques, and diagnostic instruments.

Policymakers: Give HEV prevention and control a priority in national initiatives to control infectious diseases, public health plans, and food safety laws. To lessen the effect of HEV on the health of people and the welfare of animals, allocate funds for programs of immunization, diagnosis, and surveillance.**Industry Stakeholders:** Put biosecurity measures, vaccination schedules, and hygienic standards into effect as best practices for HEV prevention and management in agricultural contexts. Encourage cooperation, traceability, and openness throughout the supply chain to guarantee food safety and customer trust.

We can meet the difficulties presented by HEV and protect the health and welfare of human and animal populations by cooperating across industries and disciplines. Let's take advantage of this chance to significantly impact the hepatitis E epidemic and create a more robust, healthy future for all.

www.ingramcontent.com/pod-product-compliance
Lightning Source LLC
Chambersburg PA
CBHW072248260726
48659CB00004BA/1476